1 MONTH OF
FREE
READING

at

www.ForgottenBooks.com

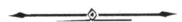

By purchasing this book you are eligible for one month membership to ForgottenBooks.com, giving you unlimited access to our entire collection of over 1,000,000 titles via our web site and mobile apps.

To claim your free month visit:

www.forgottenbooks.com/free1374677

ISBN 978-1-397-32096-4
PIBN 11374677

ADDRESS

DELIVERED BEFORE THE

American Academy of Dental Science,

AT THEIR

Thirteenth Annual Meeting,

Held in Boston, Oct. 27, 1880,

By JOSHUA TUCKER, M. D., of Boston.

Published by the Academy.

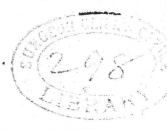

BOSTON:

S. WOODBERRY & CO, PRINTERS, 266 WASHINGTON STREET.

1881.

ADDRESS

DELIVERED BEFORE THE

American Academy of Dental Science,

AT THEIR

THIRTEENTH ANNUAL MEETING,

HELD IN BOSTON, OCT. 27, 1880,

By JOSHUA TUCKER, M. D., OF BOSTON.

PUBLISHED BY THE ACADEMY.

BOSTON:
S. WOODBERRY & CO., PRINTERS, 266 WASHINGTON STREET.
1881.

85 NEWBURY STREET, BOSTON, March 17, 1880.

JOSHUA TUCKER, M. D.,

MY DEAR DOCTOR: The committee on orator and essayist for the next annual meeting, have selected you to deliver the annual address.

Allow me to express the hope that you will comply with the desire of the committee and write an address, either on one subject, or a number of subjects.

Hoping for a favorable reply at your earliest convenience, I am,

Yours very truly,

G. T. MOFFATT,
J. T. CODMAN, } *Committee.*
C. P. WILSON,

CECIL P. WILSON,

Cor. Sec'y.

BOSTON, March 25th, 1880.

DR. CECIL P. WILSON,

MY DEAR SIR: I have received your kind note, informing me that the committee on orator and essayist have selected me to deliver the next annual address.

I am glad to serve the Academy in any manner, and I accept the invitation with pleasure.

Yours very truly,

JOSHUA TUCKER.

INTRODUCTION.

Mr. President and Gentlemen :

I desire first to acknowledge the courtesy of your committee in inviting me to speak to you, and in allowing me the privilege of selecting as many subjects for my discourse as might suit my pleasure.

Gentlemen, you are aware I have devoted myself to the study and practice of your profession nearly all my life, and in so long a period I have been obliged to consider many things which have greatly interested me; some of which I could learn from others, and some of which I could only know from my own original investigation and practical experience.

Dentistry, like the other professions, looks far back into antiquity for its origin. We have lately been given the opportunity of reading in the *Dental Cosmos* a translation of a treatise on the teeth, written by Celsus, a Roman physician, who lived eighteen hundred years ago; and in 1855, I saw at Naples, in the ancient Art Museum, some instruments taken from under the ashes of Pompeii, which, though rusty with the dampness of ages, yet bore a strong

4

resemblance, both in form and size, to those I myself had used.

Still, dentistry, as we practise it, is in most respects a child of the first half of this century. True, there have been many methods, changes and improvements since I began to study, and more may come in the future. Now, in regard to these changes, I feel as President ELIOT, of Harvard College, says in speaking of historic creeds, that " we reverence the fair and eager mind, receptive of old truths, and thankfully expectant of new."

ADDRESS.

Mr. President:

I chiefly propose to present to you to-day, some of my reasons for extracting between the years of six and twenty-one, the six-year old, or first permanent molars, when feebly organized and carious,— a subject I have always considered of the greatest importance to successful dentistry; though I may also, incidentally, offer some remarks about other matters which have interested me in an extensive practice of fifty years.

In the first place, to lay a foundation for my reasons, I consider it necessary to call your attention as briefly as possible to the organization and development of the teeth, and especially to the formative process of dentine; also, to the nature and cause of the disintegration called caries, and to say somewhat concerning the ulceration of the periosteum, and the treatment of exposed pulps.

The teeth are organized and partially developed with the alveolar process, and when they are irrupted from the gums and take their proper places in the arch, their crowns are complete shells of enamel, of normal size, length and diameter; but if *now* extracted, the *root* will be found to be a shell of dentine about half their normal length. The interior of the crown and root are filled with fibrous tissue, which extends above the shell, but in time the root elong- ates and surrounds this extended tissue, forming a shell of a complete root in length and size, with the foramen at the apex. Between the root and alveolar process is a dense, cartilaginous membrane called the periosteum. This fibrous tissue, called the pulp of the tooth, is inter- woven with arteries, veins and nerves, a fact equally evident to every practising dentist who may accidentally or carelessly wound it, by the acute pain and bleeding which follows.

The pulp is surrounded by a peculiar membraneous organization that secretes and separates the white osseous fluid, or bone element, from the red, or arterial blood, and seems also to have an inherent power or force which enables it to carry this osseous fluid to the wall surround- ing the pulp and the contiguous tissue, which becomes calcified with the wall. This calcifying process builds internally against the enamel or wall, taking in or adding to the wall, fibre after fibre, from year to year, much like the growth of a tree, layer after layer, from year to year, but externally. As this action or growth progresses from the wall inwardly, the arteries and veins of the pulp become gradually obliterated. This calcifying and obliterating process continues, if not interrupted by disease, till old age. The tissue once the pulp, now becomes entirely calcified, and healthy, solid dentine takes its place. This is the great and normal process with healthy teeth.

Now this creative action in the deposit of lime · or dentine is often deranged by a deficiency in the osseous fluid or lack of vital force, and then appear in such cases, minute cells in the body of the dentine, which can only be discovered by means of the microscope. Three years ago I read a paper at one of our evening meetings, advancing this theory, and remember with pleasure your complimentary vote to have it reread at our annual public assembly. Since that time, Dr. Frank Abbott, of New York, has intelligently and scientifically investigated dentine with the microscope, and discovered these cells, which he graphically describes as ponds. (See Cosmos., 1879.)

These cells are often formed in the earlier deposits of lime near the enamel, and within each is a nucleus of moisture which increases to a fluid that cannot evaporate or be absorbed. This fluid soon becomes morbid, and by chemical reaction generates an acid that dissolves the lime, following in the direction of the tubes till it reaches the enamel, and then attacks and perforates that. We also meet with a similar process or action in the ulceration of the periosteum by the derangement of the pulp. This may be caused by exposure, by caries or a wound from the excavator, or by anything that disrupts the surrounding membrane, allowing the red coloring matter of the arterial blood to mix with the white osseous fluid, giving the latter a red tinge, which fact may be seen in the red color of the congested crown and root. The pulp thus disturbed soon becomes morbid, and the secretions, now abnormal, are carried by the circulation through the dentine, reaching the periosteum, where in time, it produces inflammation and ulceration. Likewise, when the pulp gradually perishes in the canal, the normal circulation between the pulp and periosteum is disturbed and the action ceases; sooner or later the periosteum becomes inflamed, creates and gathers serum, which increases and changes to pus, and this generates an acrid solvent that acts on the lime, perforates the alveolar plate and soft integuments. This morbid product, in conformity with the law of all dead or effete matter in other parts of the body, is forced out externally, resulting in a fistula.

When this active solvent reaches the enamel, the disorganized dentine or decalcified tissue can be perceived within the tooth by the reflection of a mouth mirror, by a dark shade or spot through the thin or transparent enamel. In such cases, this solvent soon de-crystallizes the enamel, which becomes brittle, opaque and changed to a brown color: and if the chisel is pressed against the dark spot, the enamel scales or crumbles away and exposes the original fibrous tissue that had once been calcified dentine, but is now a decalcified, soft, and adhesive tissue, which can be removed in layers. If the excavator strikes the solid bone underneath, this will be found inflamed and very sensitive to the touch. This fibrous tissue, now decalcified and exposed, soon becomes inflamed, gangrene and decomposition follow, and the earthy matter is washed away by the saliva, leaving a cavity. Unless this is stopped by art, the vitiated fluids of the mouth act upon, and still further disintegrate the dentine, the cavity grows larger till it reaches the pulp and destroys its vital action.

I will here relate one case of the many that came under my care.

A young girl about eleven years of age, presented herself with the central incisors long, and standing a little apart. In making my examination with the mouth mirror, I discovered a dark spot within each tooth, and nearly opposite each other. I told the mother that these teeth should be filled, but believing her own eyes better, she exclaimed that the teeth were not decayed, as there was no cavity visible. I invited her to look into the mirror, and she at once perceived the dark spots. I now passed a sharp pointed instrument over the dark spots to assure her that there was still no perforation through the enamel, and explained to her the nature and probable extent of the internal decay, and the necessity of at once arresting it. After some discussion, the mother concluded to trust to my judgment. I then pressed the instrument against each tooth, in turn. The enamel crumbled easily and revealed the two cavities within, which I filled and which were no bigger than a common pin head. This and other like cases are, I think, convincing proof that such cells are often formed in the earlier deposit of dentine near the enamel.

I now turn to the cause of caries on the crowns of bicuspids and molars. These teeth are organized within the alveolar process, with a thick deposit of enamel on the points of their cusps, but this grows thinner as it advances to the centre of the grooves, where it often fails to make a perfect union, for when these teeth take their position in the jaw, for want of perfect union, we often find seams in the enamel at the centre of the grooves and indentations of the crown. In these interstices or seams, gather the acids of the saliva, which come in contact with the dentine, and so disintegration or caries begins, acting under the enamel, and when we break down the enamel to prepare the cavity for filling, we find the tissue underneath partly decomposed and often a large cavity. On removing the softened tissue, the excavator also may break through the floor of the first into another cavity beneath filled with decalcified tissue which, though sensitive to the touch, is free from decomposition. The fact of the existence of two such cavities in the same tooth, I think is convincing proof of internal as well as external derangement in its organization and growth.

External caries of the tooth, caused by the internal chemical reaction of the fluids in these cells, ponds, or interglobular spaces, can be discovered as I have said, before breakage or perforation of the enamel by a dark brown color.

External caries on the approximal surfaces of the teeth is produced by crowding and wearing during the movements of the teeth in mastication, destroying the polished surface and fracturing the crystalline strata of the enamel, and that allowing the acids of the mouth to permeate and come in contact with the dentine, and caries is the result. We can see this action by acids at the necks of the teeth, also in the indentations on the buccal surfaces of the molars when the enamel is thin or abraded.

However, I trust every dentist present has had the good fortune to see teeth so completely organized and perfect in their integrity, as to need no care on his part.

Thus far on the matter of the organization,—and the external and internal decay of the teeth.

Before I approach the subject of extraction of molars, let me, even at the risk of seeming to digress, recall something of my own experience and history as a dentist.

I began the study of dentistry fifty-three years ago, with Dr. D. C. Ambler, of Columbia, South Carolina, a skilful and genial gentleman. I continued my studies under Dr. C. Starr Brewster, meanwhile attending lectures at the South Carolina Medical College. Dr. Brewster was the pupil of Dr. Hudson, of Baltimore, who was an able and skilful dentist. I had no personal acquaintance with Dr. Hudson, but heard much of him from Dr. Brewster, who felt that to his method of filling teeth with pellets, he owed much of his own success.

·I first met Dr. Brewster in 1827, at Charleston, South Carolina, where he had gained a high reputation by many years of practice. He afterwards visited Paris, and finally settled there and became dentist to Louis Phillipe, and the royal family. He also by invitation, visited St.

Petersburg, to operate for the Emperor and his family, and was decorated with the order of St. Stanislaus, by the Czar. Dr. Brewster was the first American dentist who gained a world wide reputation in Paris. Following him are the familiar names of Dr. Evans and Dr. Gage. There were also many other dentists who gained deserved distinction in this country in the first half of the present century. Prominent, were Dr. Hayden, the first president of the first dental college in America, at Baltimore. Also, Dr. Harris, pioneer in dental literature, of the same city. In Washington, Dr. Maynard; in Philadelphia, Drs. Keocker and Fitch, each of whom published a treatise on the teeth; also, Drs. Gardette and Townsend. In New York, Drs. Eleazer Parmlee, Dodge and Trenor. Boston, Drs. Josiah Flagg, N. C. Keep, and my respected partner, Daniel Harwood, M. D. All of those gentlemen gained their reputation and success by the practice of the old method of filling teeth with pellets of soft gold, and by hand pressure.

After leaving my preceptor, Dr. Brewster, I went to Havana, Cuba, and being thrown there upon my own responsibility, I found many difficulties to overcome that tried my temper, patience and skill. I had to speak through an interpreter until I had acquired the Spanish language, and I had no English speaking dentist to consult with, and but few books.

While time thus passed away, I took my next advance by studying the nature and cause of the diseases I was called upon to treat.

I soon discovered that caries originated externally in the interstices of the enamel in the centre of the grooves of the bicuspids and molars, also where the mesial and distal surfaces came in contact and crowded.

At this time, it was my practice to fill small cavities in the center of the crowns or their indentations, and the gold would sometimes fall out. Not wishing to lose my reputation the second time, I cut away the walls and carved out the cavity and the seams, polished the surface of the dentine and waited for results. In a few years, I found that the cavities thus treated, lasted better than many I had previously filled. I therefore began to file away superficial cavities of front teeth, and polished the dentine with the same favorable result, and directed the patient to continue the friction from time to time. I have since become satisfied that friction of the dentine, stimulates the vital action of the tubulii, thereby causing a semi-vitreous deposit on the surface, which becomes nearly as hard as the enamel.

In support of this theory or principle of action, I will relate a case that recently came under my observation. A gentleman had his upper incisor teeth separated, and superficial cavities removed with the file, and the surfaces polished by Dr. Josiah Flagg of this city, fifty-one years ago. The gentleman said he had continued the polishing as directed by Dr. Flagg, and these teeth are now free from caries and doing perfect service.

Every dentist has seen this result from friction and

wearing down of the teeth in mastication. To give force to these observations I will briefly report two cases. Forty-two years ago a young lady came under my care. I extracted and filled a number of teeth. The fillings still remain in perfect service. At this time I also removed caries with a chisel from the distal side of a right superior wisdom tooth, by cutting a straight bevel from the crown to the neck of the tooth; then polished the surface, and directed the patient to continue the polishing from time to time ; and now, after a lapse of forty-two years, the chiseled surface is perfectly free from caries, and looks like polished agate. May the lady live many years, and her present dentist, whose attention has been particularly called to this case, himself report to this society the condition of these teeth at the close of half a century.

I also filled a tooth for a gentleman on the buccal surface of an under molar; and, after a time, the filling came out. I afterward carved out the cavity, leaving a straight surface from the crown to the neck of the tooth. I have not seen the gentleman for forty years, but he is now a patient of my brother, Dr. E. G. Tucker, who reports the tooth free from caries, and the surface nearly as hard as enamel.

In this connection I would also remark that I have directed the use of crystallized tannin in solution as a wash for teeth, as tannin has an affinity for the gelatine of the bone. By this chemical action the inflammation at the necks of the teeth or exposed dentine is subdued, and at the same time the gums are quieted and healed and the breath purified,

Now in relation to exposed pulps, I was in the habit of capping with lead or thin gold plate; but lead proved the more quieting and successful. The result of either case, however, was the gradual death of the pulp and finally ulceration of the periosteum. In later years I capped with oxy-chloride of zinc, a method now familiar to every dentist; but the pulp would with few exceptions gradually perish within the canal, generating a poisonous gas, which transfusing the dentine would act as a poison on the circulation of the periosteum without, and so the result would be ulceration. All credit, however, to modern dentists who think they can by treatment neutralize this poison, and restore the periosteum to health.

In my early years also I had to engraft many pivot teeth, and observed that when the pulp was extracted alive there was much less inflammation of the periosteum than when the pulp had previously and gradually perished. By the knowledge of this fact, I applied extraction to the live pulp of the roots of such front teeth as I thought judicious to fill.

My method in such cases, was to enlarge the place of exposure, and pass a barbed broach quickly to the end of the canal, when with a slight turn of the instrument, the pulp was excised and readily extracted. If the removal of the pulp was attended with bleeding, I treated the canal a few days with creosote, but if free from bleeding, I prepared the canal at once for filling, gaining better access to it by perforating the palatal surface of the enamel sufficiently to press the gold directly to the apex of the root. By this method, I have had many crowns last twenty-five or more years.

A front tooth, however, whose root had a dead pulp and fistula, I prepared for filling by opening freely into the canal to enable me to extirpate perfectly, all carious or diseased dentine, and carry the pellets of soft gold free and direct to the apex and wall of the root, great care being taken to completely stop or seal the foramen. The result was generally the healing of the fistula, and final restoration of the periosteum to comparative health.

The extraction of a live pulp was at that time considered heroic treatment, and my associate, Dr. Harwood, would comfort his patients with the remark, that although it might be painful, it was nevertheless scientific practice; but now in these days, with ether or gas, the extraction of a live nerve becomes an easy and painless operation, bringing but little inconvenience to the patient, and much more durability to the root; at the same time, the periosteum is much less likely to ulcerate. I *have* devitalized the pulps with arsenic, but was always doubtful of the effect on the periosteum.

Now with regard to extraction of molars. In my first years of practice I separated front teeth for filling with a file, but found that in a few years they would approach and become carious around the gold. My next advance was to file wider spaces, leaving a shoulder at the necks of the contiguous teeth, hoping thus to prevent the crowding. I also separated bicuspids and molars with a chisel or file, making a wide space of the V form. With this practice I was more successful. Still they would at times approach and result in the recurrence of caries around the gold.

Studying now to still further overcome these difficulties, I decided to extract the six-year, or first permanent molars, if diseased, but experience soon taught me that I sometimes extracted them too early, as I found the alveolus would quickly absorb, and the second molar the sooner make its appearance and pitch forward, and I would thus lose the object I hoped to gain. My last advance was to wait until the second molars were erupted, and had taken their positions, and were well rooted, then to extract the six-year old, or first permanent molars, when carious.

In time I had the satisfaction of seeing the bicuspids fall back to the molars, and to give relief to the former crowding. I could often see the good results of this practice even to the centre of the arch. Exceptions to this rule of extracting the first molars occurred when the second molar or second bicuspid were the more carious. It being a fact that teeth become carious where they touch and crowd, the remedy should be self-evident.

_____

Having adopted this treatment of judicious removal just described, as time went on I further discovered, agreeably and much to my surprise, that the molars and bicuspid teeth on either side of the one that was extracted had changed their character; that the dentine had become more dense, less sensitive to the touch of the excavator, and more durable when filled.

The observant dentist has doubtless recognized the fact that when a molar stands alone in the jaw it becomes more dense and durable when filled, and the alveolar process also become solidified around the isolated tooth.

The agriculturist understands when the fruit on his trees or vines is too thick and feebly organized, that in order to obtain a full and healthy growth he must use his pruning knife, well knowing that every particle of nourishment developed for the many will now be utilized by the few. And Shakespeare remarks:

> " All superficial branches lop away,
> That bearing boughs may live."

Another has also observed : " The knife that amputates is often the only means of preservation of physical life."

Following these laws as regards the growth and health of young teeth, I have practised on the principle of *judicious* pruning. While I have used my utmost skill to preserve the eight anterior teeth of either jaw, it has been my practice to extract back of the first bicuspids such teeth as had exposed pulps, unless very important for use. As I have before said, if the surrounding membrane of the pulp is exposed, disrupted and bleeds, the pulp is sure to perish, and sooner or later be followed by ulceration of the periosteum.

Pathology has taught me that the continued oozing of dead or effete matter from one or more chronic fistulæ into the mouth, and taken into the stomach of children, or even adults, must prove injurious to general health; but our wise mother, Nature, in time removes all such dead teeth and roots regardless of modern theories.

I have also extracted devitalized teeth and roots, so that the periosteum of such teeth and roots shall not absorb or appropriate that nourishment or osseous element, which would be better utilized by those remaining. Likewise I have observed, when the six-year-old molars had been extracted, the osseous element created for the extracted teeth seemed to be carried to and utilized by the growing wisdom teeth. Then when these teeth make their appearance they have become highly organized and developed, large and dense, and fill the space at the angle of the jaw, and prove useful in after life. But I desire it to be understood that when the first and second molars are perfectly developed and free from caries, and the wisdom teeth are small and feebly developed, and crowded out of line at the angle of the jaw, they were extracted, giving relief to the crowding of the remaining molars, and I could see good results coming from this practice.

———

Concerning the growth of the teeth from the enamel inwardly, and that of the vegetable from the center outwardly, they have as before intimated correspondent phenomena in their self-acting and self-producing power.

———

I have listened to discussions on this subject by gentlemen of this Academy and elsewhere, who expressed opinions differing entirely from mine. The arguments advanced by many, however, seemed to rest on the assumption that by extracting so many teeth the jaw would thereby contract, and so produce hereditary results, which would prove unfortunate to children and grandchildren. I would only say in reply to such opinions that I have looked about for other and similar hereditary physical results, with other organs of children and grandchildren, and as yet have entirely and completely failed of success.

Let me illustrate: A short time ago, while walking on Boston Common, I *interviewed,* somewhat after the fashion of the day, a stranger, who was a cripple, with one leg and a crutch. Among other things the gentleman said that he moved about with comfort and without difficulty; that he had made five trips to Europe; that he lost his limb at fourteen years of age, and at twenty-one could jump a bar as high as any of his companions: also that what was once the strength of both limbs now seemed to be transferred and centered in the remaining *one.* I did not ask the gentleman if he had conferred a crutch and one leg upon each of his children through hereditary law; that remains for my intelligent friends, and all such as have any doubt, what his answer would be.

Finally, though I have considered that much of my professional success has been due to the early adoption of this system, relating to the extraction of six-year-old molars, yet it must be remembered, as I have before observed, that my practice in this regard was modified if the second molars or second bicuspids were more feeble and diseased. The observant dentist of course will be governed by the peculiar state of the mouth, and conditions of the teeth, for it is manifest, no *one* treatment will answer for all cases.

Further, I have been governed by a strong desire to give as much comfort as possible during youth, but not to the detriment and expense of the future. Therefore the object and aim of my practice was to save a sufficient number of teeth for looks, as well as for healthy and comfortable use to middle and old age. And when in active practice, having charge of a child's mouth with feeble and diseased teeth, I considered that if by removing a few I could the better retain the many, even to the number of twenty-eight or twenty-four teeth, I had attained the maximum of my professional success.

———————

Mr. President, I trust these remarks have not been so extended as to weary you, and that I have not seemed to be too tenacious of my own theories. Every science and every art has its laws and its limitations, and every special case too has its special peculiarities.

It is by ascertaining what law applies to each case that the best results can be attained. This should be the work of every thoughtful dentist to understand thoroughly the nature of teeth, the laws of growth, disease and death. Thus we can intelligently assist nature in her struggle to remove devitalized teeth and roots, and by art restore those remaining to health.

I have striven to impress upon all younger men with whom I have been brought in contact, that *judgment* and *discretion must* be used by each one for himself, but that no judgment or discretion is valuable, except so far as it is founded upon knowledge, and that can only be gained by study, thought and experience. Finally, I ask you to take what I have said, think of it, to consider for yourselves how far it is correct, and to follow it only as you may find it based on true information and just reasoning.